I0101470

Diabetes:
Its Cause and Its Treatment With Insulin
By
Russell M. Wilder

Copyright © 2024 by BTBPUBLISHING.COM

All rights reserved. No part of this publication may be reproduced or transmitted in any form or by any means electronic or mechanical, including information storage and retrieval systems without permission in writing from the publisher, except for student research using the appropriate citations.

ISBN: 978-1-63652-281-4

DIABETES

ITS CAUSE AND ITS TREATMENT WITH INSULIN

RUSSELL M. WILDER

CONTENTS

INTRODUCTION

W hen the scientific body that awards the Nobel prize each year met to consider the award for 1923, there was no question or debate as to the discovery that merited the honor. The prize was granted to Doctors F. G. Banting and J. J. R. MacLeod of Toronto for their work in the discovery of insulin, and each immediately donated one-half the award to colleagues who had shared in this discovery, Doctors C. H. Best and J. B. Collip.

In November, 1920, Dr. Banting, who had returned from war service, was practicing medicine in London, Ontario, and was demonstrating physiology in the medical school of Western University at that place. While reading an article in a surgical magazine, he chanced on a sentence which aroused the train of thought that finally led to his discovery of insulin—a substance that means a longer and more satisfactory life to diabetics.

The article which he read concerned a gland, known as the pancreas, that lies close to the stomach and the upper part of the intestines. This gland is composed of two portions, one of which creates a juice poured into the intestine, which aids in the digestion of food; it is the external secretion and it contains trypsin and two other digestive ferments. The pancreas contains also certain cells which, when seen through the microscope, are marked off from the remaining tissue and which are known by the peculiar name "Islands of Langerhans," the latter being the name of their discoverer.

Diabetes centuries old.—Now diabetes is no new disease.

It was described by Aretaeus, a Greek who lived in the third century, A.D., and hundreds of scientists have worked steadily on the problem ever since that time. Indeed the history of the discovery of insulin is typical of all great medical discoveries of modern times. It represents the summation of a vast amount of knowledge contributed bit by bit by scientists all over the world. When Banting conceived his idea, he took it to Dr. MacLeod, director of physiologic research in the University of Toronto. Professor MacLeod, seeing the possibilities in the investigation, gave him opportunity to work, and provided him with a young assistant, Dr. C. H. Best. The particular problem on which they were to work was the extraction from the pancreas of another secretion, an internal secretion, not poured by the pancreas through a special duct into any other organ or to the exterior, but going instead into the blood stream.

Pancreas yields substance.—Previous investigations had indicated that this secretion was manufactured in the Islands of Langerhans. It was known that when the tube which carries the external secretion—trypsin—was tied, the trypsin would back up into the pancreas, and by its digestive action would destroy the glandular tissue, leaving an organ which consisted chiefly of island tissue.

The investigators did such an operation on a dog. It was also known that an animal might be made diabetic by removing the pancreas; this operation was performed on another dog. Then, when sufficient time had elapsed to permit the breaking down of the pancreas in the first animal, it was painlessly chloroformed, the pancreas removed and an extract made from it. The extract consisted chiefly of island tissue, and this extract was injected into the diabetic dog. The result was the discovery that such injections produced a lower amount of sugar in the dog's blood and in its urine. This and similar experiments established positively the fact that there was present within the pancreas, and quite certainly in the island tissue chiefly, some substance, not available in the body of the diabetic, which was capable of meeting a deficiency and aiding the diabetic to make proper use of sugar.

Drug dosage and animal experiments.—It now became necessary to devise a method of obtaining the extract in such form as to permit injections into the human being without danger from poisoning by extraneous and unnecessary substances, in other words, a pure product. It also became necessary to devise a method for measuring the dose to be given. How many persons who receive a dose of a medicine realize the amount of investigation necessary to determine these factors? It is necessary to test the effects of a drug on animals before it can be tried on the human being, and it is necessary to study very carefully the changes in the body following the administration of the drug, in order to be certain that no undesirable actions occur.

The Canadian investigators worked in a wholly scientific manner. Their experiments show great attention to the matter of controls. For each animal that was tested, there was a normal animal with which to compare it. The investigators used many dogs, and a vast number of rabbits in making these necessary tests. Not until all the factors of danger had been thoroughly controlled was the drug administered to man. Had it been given without the guiding knowledge obtained by the observations on rabbits, it seems certain that overdoses might have been administered and patients have died.

Overdose of insulin dangerous.—The effects of an overdose of insulin are striking; there is too great a lowering of the amount of sugar, and severe convulsions ensue which may lead to death. Insulin is a powerful remedy; its effects are certain and accurately measurable. If a human being is given too much, his blood sugar falls to a lower concentration. When he gets it around 0.07 per cent he begins to be anxious and nervous about himself. He is likely to become pale, or to flush and perspire profusely. If the blood sugar concentration goes still lower his speech may become disturbed, and he may even manifest mental disturbances. These things too may be prevented, and immediately stopped once they have ensued, by the giving of a small amount of sugar, as for example in the form of four to eight ounces of orange juice. These facts also were discovered by properly conducted experiments.

The investigators now turned their attention to the problem of this disease in human beings, and the results have already been broadcasted through medical periodicals, newspapers and magazines. They are far beyond the early hopes of scientific investigators of the disease. In that terminal stage of diabetes known as coma, when the patient sinks into unconsciousness, insulin seems actually to restore life. Of far greater importance, it offers for the vast majority of diabetics comfort and extended existence. Its administration is closely bound with a knowledge of the food taken into the body, for it is known that a certain amount of insulin will aid the body in handling a certain amount of sugar. When the physician decides to place his patient on the insulin treatment, he usually asks that the patient come into a hospital so that he may first find out the patient's normal ability to digest sugar, and it is this ability that the physician supplements by the giving of insulin.

Manufacture and sale.—One of the unusual aspects of the insulin discovery was the method of control in its sale. The discoverers did not wish to profit unduly by their work, but they were anxious that its manufacture and application on a large scale be scientifically controlled. Arrangements were therefore made to have it manufactured under accurate supervision in the United States by the Eli Lilly Company, and in Canada by the Connaught Laboratories, and more recently in certain other home and foreign laboratories.

The process of manufacture is an interesting one. The Islands of Langerhans constitute a small portion of what is relatively a small gland. In stock yards and packing houses this gland is called sweet breads; the sweet breads served under glass in the restaurants are usually the pancreas of the sheep or hog, since these are small. The beef pancreas is a much larger organ, weighing about a pound or a pound and a half.

The method devised by Collip for obtaining insulin from the pancreas involves repeated extraction of the ground-up pancreas with alcohol, in order to remove the unnecessary tissue substances. When this is done on a small scale in the chemical laboratory, there is, of course, considerable wastage of raw material and of substances used in the extraction.

The application of the matter on a commercial scale involved additional problems. They were not only overcome successfully, but continued improvements have made possible the provision of the life-saving remedy at a reasonable price.

Juvenile diabetes.—One of the most striking effects of the work was the result of the use of the remedy in the diabetes of children, or juvenile diabetics. This condition had previously been considered invariably fatal. Now the child may be treated satisfactorily, and it seems possible that its development under the influence of the drug may permit a gradual lowering of the dosage to amounts that may be administered with little expense or difficulty.

After the investigators had completed the trials of the preparation in their own hospital, plans were made for extensive clinical investigation in other institutions in which there were men capable of conducting scientific studies on diabetes. More than 50 institutions were utilized in order to give the drug the most complete possible scientific trial before offering it to the medical profession in general; and when at last these trials were completed and the co-operating manufacturing concerns had fully developed the machinery for production of the drug on a large scale, it was released to the medical profession throughout the world.

Patients must do their part.—It should be understood that if the patient is to receive the greatest benefit from this new remedy, he must co-operate fully and intelligently with his physician. As soon as he discovers through competent examination that he is excreting sugar in his urine, he should consult his physician as to the use of the drug and a proper diet.

In many instances, the use of insulin is unnecessary because the patient is able to live satisfactorily without insulin on a diet with the proper amount of sugar or carbohydrate material. In other instances, the dosage of insulin may be very small, but this will depend on a careful and intelligent study of each case.

It is now rather generally known by the public that insulin is a preparation which is administered hypodermically, that is, injected with a needle under the skin. It cannot be taken by mouth, because the substance is digested before it can be absorbed into the blood. This does not mean that the patient must seek his physician for every treatment, because many competent specialists in the treatment of this disease have found that patients may be taught to regulate their diet and use the drug intelligently.

Recognition of the work.—As soon as it became known that this discovery was available, diabetics flocked to their physicians and began to inquire as to the possibilities of its use to "cure" the disease; but the drug is not in the usual sense of the word a "cure" for diabetes. Diabetes represents the absence from the body, probably as the result of disease, of certain substances which are responsible for the control of the digestion and use of sugar, and insulin cannot restore these tissues or substances any more than the injections of other glands can restore youth to the aged. It can only replace temporarily the substances that are absent; but in the case of a diabetic, this constitutes the difference between life and death.

Naturally Doctors Banting, Best, Collip and MacLeod have received great honors at the hands of their colleagues and of the world. The Canadian government has granted to Dr. Banting the sum of $7,500 per year for life; the Ontario government has provided $10,000 a year for a chair of medical research, now held for the first time by Dr. Banting; learned societies throughout the world have greeted him with the applause usually accorded only to military heroes.

The victor in the conflict of science with disease is certainly deserving of the wreath of the conqueror.

MORRIS FISHBEIN.

DIABETES: ITS CAUSE AND ITS TREATMENT WITH INSULIN

*I*nsulin a welcome discovery.—The discovery of a method for obtaining insulin in a form suitable for use in treating diabetes is a cause for genuine rejoicing. The sensational newspaper and magazine articles that greeted the discovery were, in a sense, a public expression of such rejoicing, and their exaggerations may be forgiven if this is remembered. The effort to gain an understanding and a sure method of controlling diabetes has taken years, and while the scientist delved in his laboratory, the seemingly unconquerable disease continued to take an ever-increasing toll of young and aged victims. In New York City, for instance, where statistics collected by Dr. Emerson are most reliable, the deaths from diabetes in 1866 were only 1 for each 2,437 deaths from all causes. In 1923, one death in every fifty-one was due to diabetes. The diabetic death rate in New York City was trebled between 1880 and 1920 for ages up to forty-five years. For ages of forty-five and more, it was quintupled. There are probably more than a million patients with diabetes in the United States. No wonder then that mankind in general was overjoyed when the news came that the young Canadians, Banting and Best, had discovered insulin.

Russell M. Wilder

THE NATURE OF DIABETES

*D*iabetes a disorder of metabolism. —What is this insulin and what does it do? Before this is answered, the nature of the chemical disorder that is called diabetes must be somewhat understood, and to supply this understanding, a partial review of the chemistry and physiology of nutrition must be made.

The processes of life are largely chemical. The warmth of the body is provided by combustion, oxidation of food. If the supply of food is discontinued, life ends, and the body cools exactly as a gasoline motor stops and cools off when its supply of fuel is exhausted. Similarly, if the machinery for transforming food into energy is impaired, life will lag. This is what happens in diabetes; the disorder is much like that of a motor which misses fire when its ignition system is out of order. Food, like gasoline, contains energy, and life results from the conversion of this potential energy into body heat and muscular activity. The processes involved in this conversion are spoken of collectively as "metabolism." Diabetes is a disorder of metabolism. There are other disorders of metabolism, but none so common as that of diabetes.

Carbohydrate, protein and fat. —The food supply of mankind is limited to the tissues of plants and animals, and the fuel in all such foods is either a carbohydrate, a fat, or a protein. Carbohydrates are starches and sugars; fats are oils, lards and complex materials such as may be found in brain, and egg yolk; protein is abundant in lean meat and cheese. Compared to the protein, the carbohydrates and fats are relatively simple chemical substances, fairly stable and, hence, easy to study chemically. Proteins are excessively changeable, to which character they owe their name. Some proteins are called albumins. Egg albumin, egg white, is a typical protein possessing all of the essential protein characteristics. The carbohydrates and fats serve chiefly as fuels, while the proteins, besides providing energy, build or rebuild the living tissues of the body. A diet may be deficient in either fat or carbohydrate, and still remain adequate. It must, however, provide a modicum of protein, since parts of the protoplasmic machinery of the tissues are constantly wearing out and requiring replacement.

Foods are disintegrated by catalysts.—While the conversion of the energy in carbohydrates, fats and proteins into the life flame is a process of combustion or oxidation, it is not a simple burning or explosion, as in the case of the fuel ignited in the cylinder of the gasoline motor, but proceeds by successive steps or stages. The earliest of these steps is taken in the kitchen where food is prepared by cooking. There the starches are softened and partly broken up, and the proteins are coagulated. The next stages are passed during digestion, beginning in the mouth, where the ptyalin, a ferment in the salivary juice, attacks starches, and continuing as the food passes successively through the stomach and the intestine. Ferments are also called catalysts. At each and every stage of digestion and assimilation some catalyst facilitates and accelerates the process of decomposition in a manner similar to the action of ptyalin on starch, or of yeast in brewing beer. Consequently, the food, before it has descended more than half way down the length of the small intestine, has been disintegrated chemically into fragments that are smaller and, chemically, much less complex than the original foodstuffs. The starches are split into sugars, the chief of which is glucose; the fats are broken into fatty acid and glycerin; the proteins are torn apart and comparatively simpler structures, the so-called amino-acids, result.

Sugar in the blood.—The food fragments resulting from digestion are soaked up through the intestinal wall into the blood and lymph, both of which fluids circulate freely around the intestine, and in the blood and lymph they can always be found, if suitable chemical means are adopted for detecting them. They are abundant in the blood during the hours following meal-taking, and diminish in fasting. The sugar glucose, for instance, is present in blood taken early in the morning in a concentration of about one part in each thousand, or 0.1 per cent, but when carbohydrates are being digested, one and one-half parts of glucose in each thousand, or 0.15 per cent are found.

The rôle of the liver.—The next stages of metabolism occur in the liver, to which the blood passes immediately after leaving the intestine. Here is a veritable chemical laboratory wherein innumerable transformations are worked. Some of them are now understood, and here, as later elsewhere, at every step of change, a catalyst is present to facilitate each separate chemical alteration. Many catalysts are very specific, accomplishing one definite task; others are more generally active. They have been likened to keys, which, fitting into certain locks, permit the locks to be turned. Without these catalysts or accelerators, transformations would occur so slowly that active life, such as ours, would be impossible.

In the liver much of the sugar is removed from the blood and organized into a starch-like substance called glycogen. Thus stored, it is available later, when the blood may be poor in sugar. One of the main functions of the liver is to maintain a nearly constant concentration of sugar in the blood, which it does by subtracting sugar whenever, as after meals, the blood stream is flooded, and adding sugar at those times between meals, and at night, when the sugar level in the blood is low.

In the liver, the amino-acid fragments of proteins are partly destroyed, ammonia is split off from them and changes into a waste product, urea, which is later excreted by the kidneys. Also sugar is made from many of the fragments of protein, and this sugar is either stored away as glycogen with the sugar originating from carbohydrate, or added to the blood. Nearly 60 per cent, by dry weight, of the protein eaten is thus changed to sugar, and as a final result of the normal processes of digestion, and action of the liver, we find that all of the carbohydrate, approximately 58 per cent of the protein, and it is supposed, 10 per cent of the fat of the food, eventually finds its way into sugar.

If we desire to know how much sugar a certain food will add to the metabolism, that is, the sugar value of the food, we must know both the weight of the food and how much of this weight is carbohydrate, how much is protein, and how much is fat. The sugar value will be the sum obtained by adding the weight of the carbohydrate, 58 per cent of the weight of the protein, and 10 per cent of the weight of the fat. For instance, a slice of bread weighing 2 ounces or 60 gm., spread with one-third of an ounce or 10 gm. of butter would be 32 gm. of carbohydrate, 6 gm. of protein and 11 gm. of fat. The sugar value of this mixture would be 32 plus 3.5 plus 1.1 or 36.6 gm. A glass of whole milk, 6 ounces or 180 gm. of milk, would contain 9 gm. of carbohydrate, 5 gm. of protein and 7 gm. of fat, and its sugar value would be 9 plus 3 plus 0.7, or nearly 13 gm.

After passing the liver, the blood enters the heart which then pumps it throughout the system of tubes called arteries into all the crevices of the body. Every tissue is thus bathed constantly with circulating fluids which contain sugar and the other elements of nutrition in forms suitable for utilization.

The liberation of energy in the tissues.—In the blood itself, no important chemical transformation occurs. The food fragments are picked out of the blood by the tissues and in the living protoplasms of each tissue, those important changes occur which constitute the most essential processes of life. These are, first, the building up of new protoplasmic matter, namely, growth and tissue repair, and, second, the liberation of energy by further decomposition and final burning or oxidation. Again each step of transformation requires the aid of some energizer or catalyst. The presence of many of these catalysts is only surmised. Some of them, however, have been captured and their mysteries are exposed. Among these is thyroxin, which Kendall showed to be the chief product of the thyroid gland. Thyroxin sets the pace of life. The rate of oxygen utilization is governed largely by it, so that when the thyroid gland is destroyed or not functioning, as in some forms of goiter, energy transformation proceeds at a slower tempo.

Insulin a catalyst.—We come now to diabetes, a condition which results from the lack or deficiency of a catalyst called insulin. The function of insulin, it seems, is to prepare sugar for utilization.

Diabetes a lack of insulin.—In diabetes, sugar escapes utilization in whole or in part. As it circulates normally in the blood, it is locked up, so to speak, and is unavailable either for storage as glycogen, or for oxidation or other transformation. Its energy is sealed, and before it becomes available a lock must be turned. The key to this lock is insulin, and in the absence of this key the normal means by which sugar is removed from the blood are unavailing, and in consequence, the level of sugar in the blood rises, and sugar appears in the urine.

Symptoms of diabetes.—The symptoms of diabetes are due for the greater part to the accumulation in the blood and excretion in the urine of unused sugar. On leaving the body, sugar carries water with it. A diabetic patient may pass many quarts of urine daily. This is a phenomenon like the drying of meats or fish by salting them. Water is subtracted in such amounts that the body dries; even the skin becomes dry, and the tongue may cleave to the roof of the mouth. Furthermore, much otherwise available food energy is lost with sugar in the urine. As much as a pound of sugar may be passed in a day. Consequently, the tissues starve in the midst of plenty. The appetite, therefore, is sharpened, but the more the patient eats, the greater becomes the wastage of food energy, and the more severe the symptoms.

Acid poisoning.—This is not all or, by any means, the worst. It so happens that fat, which under suitable circumstances, is readily metabolized, fails to oxidize smoothly when less than a certain minimum of sugar is being used. The fats, it is said, burn in the fire of carbohydrates. If a perfectly normal person is deprived of carbohydrate and fed only fat and a little protein, certain products of incompleted combustion of fat will accumulate in the body. These substances are acetone, aceto-acetic acid, and the hydroxybutyric acid. Acetone is not very poisonous, nor is hydroxybutyric acid, but aceto-acetic acid behaves somewhat after the manner of the anesthetics like chloroform. If a person has diabetes of some severity, acetone bodies may arise even when carbohydrate is fed because only *burning* sugar prevents their formation, and in severe diabetes the carbohydrates fail to burn.

Diabetic coma.—In diabetes, therefore, such amounts of aceto-acetic acid may be formed that the patient is actually anesthetized and falls into unconsciousness. This is diabetic coma, which in the past has been the chief cause of death in the diabetes of children and young persons. The proper use of insulin should prevent these deaths from coma.

THE STORY OF INSULIN

M *inkowski's discovery.*—The story of insulin began a generation ago with the discovery of German investigators, Minkowski and von Mehring. This was in 1889, and until then the relation of the pancreas to diabetes was scarcely suspected, and no one had an idea where to look for the means to check the disease. The pancreas is an organ about the size of one's hand which pours digestive juices into the intestine.

Removal of pancreas causes diabetes.—Minkowski was studying digestion and it happened in the course of certain investigations, that it became necessary to operate on a dog and remove this organ. A few days later it was noticed that flies were attracted in great numbers by the urine of this dog. The urine was examined, and the reason for the flies and the relation of the pancreas to diabetes was at once apparent. The urine contained sugar. Another animal was operated on, the pancreas removed and diabetes followed. Cats, swine, and frogs were then experimented with. In every case, complete removal of the pancreas resulted in severe diabetes, while partial removal caused a more chronic and milder diabetes.

The islands of Langerhans.—Previously, in 1869, Paul Langerhans, described peculiar clumps or islands of cells which differ in appearance from the bulk of the tissue in the pancreas. In 1890, Scobolew and Schulze showed that if the ducts leading from the pancreas were tied off, the islands withstood the destruction that was wrought in the rest of the organ by backing up of the pancreatic secretions. Animals treated in this manner did not develop diabetes, and it was concluded, therefore, that it was the islands that manufactured the anti-diabetic material of the pancreas. The name "insulin" was suggested for this material in 1916 by an Englishman, Shafer.

Previous attempts to obtain insulin.—In the meantime, efforts were being made by numerous scientists to extract from the pancreas the anti-diabetic principle. Some of these attempts nearly succeeded. Many of them failed because it was not known then that insulin is rendered inactive when it is given by mouth and subjected to the disintegrating action of the juices in the digestive tract. Innumerable attempts were made to control diabetes by feeding either fresh pancreas, or pills and pellets manufactured from the pancreas. Thus far, all such efforts have been in vain, and yet various drug companies continue to sell pancreatic pills as diabetic remedies. The results obtained by grafting pieces of pancreas into dogs previously made diabetic by the removal of the pancreas have been more successful. The experimental diabetes of animals so treated can be controlled, but such procedures offer nothing to mankind, because grafts made from a lower animal to man invariably atrophy, that is, shrink up and disappear.

Banting's idea.—Thus the subject stood when, in the autumn of 1920, Frederick Banting, recently home from the war, began his work. The idea came, he writes, while reading an article dealing with the relation of the islands of Langerhans to diabetes. In his own words, it was this: "From the passage in this article, which gives a resumé of degenerative changes in the acini (cells connected with the ducts or passageway system) of the pancreas following ligation of the ducts, the idea presented itself that since the acinous, but not the islet tissue, degenerates after this operation, advantage might be taken of this fact to prepare an active extract of islet tissue. The subsidiary hypothesis was that trypsinogen (one of the digestive ferments prepared by the acinous cells) or its derivatives was antagonistic to the internal secretion of the gland. The failures of other investigators in this much worked field were thus accounted for." In other words, the failure of his predecessors, Banting thought, was due to the probability that the digestive juices of the pancreas destroyed insulin before it could be extracted from the islands, and his plan was to circumvent this difficulty by first destroying the part of the pancreas concerned in making these juices.

The first insulin.—Banting took his idea to Professor Macleod of the

THE CAUSE OF DIABETES

*D*isease of the pancreas a cause of diabetes.—The pancreas, whose removal Minkowski showed caused diabetes, is located in the abdomen near the stomach and pours its digestive juices through a channel or duct into the intestine. The organ has a second function, as has been told above, namely, to make insulin. This second product, which is elaborated by the islands of Langerhans, goes into the blood. The Langerhans islands are properly regarded as a distinct and separate organ. They are, however, so intimately associated and intermingled with the rest of the pancreas that any disease or injury of the pancreas may affect them seriously, reduce their insulin-making capacity and thus cause diabetes. Actually a large part of the pancreas may be destroyed before diabetes results. In dogs, little more than one-tenth of the gland remaining intact is sufficient to prevent the excretion of sugar. Men are more susceptible to diabetes than dogs, but even in men the pancreas may be seriously affected by inflammation or cancer before its insulin capacity is reduced to the point where actual insulin shortage is manifest.

The body is so constructed that every organ has a factor of safety. A very large amount of the liver, for instance, can be diseased before any failure in its function is detectable. The same is true of the kidneys and of the heart, and the factor of safety in the case of the pancreas explains why we do not all have diabetes. Very few people have a normal pancreas, because inflammations in organs near the pancreas are fairly common; for instance, inflammation of the gallbladder, and very frequently the pancreas is involved in such inflammation. However, the number of persons with known gallbladder disease who develop diabetes, is not appreciably greater than that of persons without any evidence of such inflammations.

Hardening of arteries a cause of diabetes.—The pancreas may be injured, as is true of all of the organs of the body, by disturbance of its blood supply, especially through hardening of the walls of the arterial tubes which bring it its blood, and narrowing of their lumens or passageways. Older persons with hardened arteries may develop diabetes in this manner. On the other hand, many persons have extreme arterial disease and consequent destruction of pancreatic islands without diabetes.

Infections a cause of diabetes.—The delicate tissues of the pancreas, just as in the case of other organs, may be poisoned in the course of a general disease, such as scarlet fever, mumps, or influenza and, in consequence, diabetes may result from such diseases. There is, however, nothing specific in this. A certain number of cases of diabetes can be traced to a preceding acute intoxication of this character, but it is by no means true that any one of the known infections is always followed by diabetes.

Functional overstrain the chief cause of diabetes.—Functional overstrain is a recognized cause of disease, especially of the heart, but also of other organs. The heart may be irreparably injured by excessive exertion. Functional overstrain of the pancreatic islands resulting from long continued overeating is a cause of much diabetes. Persons who persistently overeat are usually markedly overweight. Some thin people are also equally prone to overeat, and yet, for some thus far unknown reason, remain thin.

Obesity a mark of overeating and functional overstrain of the pancreas.—The rule, however, is that overeating leads to obesity, and it is a well known fact that many diabetic patients are, or have been, overweight. Dr. Joslin, for instance, found among 1,000 diabetic patients, 75 per cent who either were, or had been, over normal weight. Dr. Joslin says that it takes ten diabetic patients to make a ton of diabetes. Overeating with attendant long continued functional overstrain of Langerhans islands is probably the most common of all causes of diabetes.

Sugar eating.—It is of considerable significance that the increasing incidence of diabetes in America is coincident with the enormous increase in the sugar consumption. In the decade 1880 to 1890, the annual sugar consumption was 44 pounds per capita. In 1921, it had risen to 84 pounds, and in 1922 to 103 pounds. The death rate for diabetes in 1890 was 5.5 for each 100,000; in 1921, it was 16.8 for each 100,000. It is easier to overeat of sugar than of almost any other food known, and it is probable that sugar imposes a greater functional strain on the pancreas than do the starches or fats. Starches swell up and fill the stomach readily, thus checking the appetite; furthermore they are slowly absorbed into the blood. Sugar goes into solution, passes the stomach quickly, is absorbed almost instantly and at once demands attention from the pancreas. The common desserts are sweets. When we are glutted with meat and potatoes, we still have room for sweets and we can always find room for candies. The rage for soft drinks since the abolition of alcoholic beverages is certain to increase the crop of new cases of diabetes. I have seen several patients who have been suddenly precipitated into an extreme stage of diabetes and coma by a soft drink spree.

Diabetes may occur without provocation.—Not infrequently, among younger persons and children, diabetes appears out of a clear sky with apparently no provoking cause. No inflammation has occurred in the pancreas of these patients, so far as any good evidence shows; they are young and therefore not afflicted with arterial disease, and they have never been overweight and have not overeaten. How can we explain the diabetes of these children and young persons, and how can we explain why some fat persons and not all escape diabetes, and why some patients with very little disease of their pancreas have diabetes and others with very extensive destruction of the pancreas do not have it?

Heredity of the tendency to diabetes.—The answer, probably, lies in the more or less shadowy realm of heredity. Some of us are born with weak eyes and others with weak islands, and the degree of original island weakness determines the susceptibility of the islands both to functional overstrain from overeating and to injury from infectious diseases or from poor circulation of the blood. If the diabetic tendency of an individual is marked, diabetes may develop, in very early life. The pancreas here is too weak to withstand the normal functional strain of growth. When this is the case, the disease is of extreme severity. If the diabetic tendency is slight, it may not show itself except as the result of long continued overeating. If the pancreatic islands are functionally strong, they withstand infections and injury from disease or poor blood supply; if weak, they fail and diabetes results. Diabetes rather infrequently occurs in several members of the same family, but the fact that this happens rather infrequently does not mean that the tendency fails to pass by heredity. Many persons who are considered normal may have this tendency without showing any evidence of it throughout life.

THE TREATMENT OF DIABETES

*P**revention.*—A stitch in time will save nine diabetic patients. Typhoid, small-pox, diphtheria, yellow fever and a number of other diseases have been practically eliminated. Tuberculosis, otherwise known as the white plague, is rapidly being chained. Why not do the same with diabetes? We have seen that overeating is the common cause. Let us, therefore, teach the virtues of keeping lean and fit. Incidentally, such teaching may help to control other chronic diseases. There is reason to believe that heart trouble, high blood pressure, gallstone and cancer, occur in the obese with greater frequency than in the lean. Obesity is a mark of long continued functional overstrain of all the organs of the body. Overeating of carbohydrates and proteins is especially injurious to the pancreas. In Berlin, during the war when the food supplies of the populace were greatly reduced and sugar and meat in particular were scarce, the number of new patients with diabetes decreased immensely. In America, with growing luxury and rising sugar consumption, diabetes is increasing by leaps and bounds. The Jews, as a race, have much diabetes, not because they are Jews, but because so many of them are luxury lovers, overeaters, and fat Jews. Diabetes cannot be entirely eliminated by preventing overeating. As we have seen, thin people are not immune if the heredity tendency in them is strong; and they develop the severest form of diabetes at a relatively tender age, and yet it is possible that even the number of these may be reduced in time. A leading authority once published the family trees of a number of diabetic families and these family trees suggest that the tendency to diabetes becomes stronger with each succeeding generation. In the grandparents the disease was mild and came on late in life—not until they had overeaten, presumably, for many years and were fat. In the parents the disease was more severe and appeared earlier in life, the result, presumably, of less overeating. In the third generation, the disease occurred in the children with still less provocation from overeating. Perhaps we can save our grandchildren, therefore, by keeping ourselves fit, and thus stamp out the diabetes of childhood which is always severe and, therefore, the most dreaded. It is worth a trial.

Detection of early cases.—Doctor Joslin, who has done more than anyone else to teach the diabetic people of America how to keep well and strong, urges that everyone have the urine tested annually on his or her birthday. Life insurance examinations, are now fortunately much more frequent than formerly, and reveal numerous early cases of diabetes. Diabetic patients, who have been properly treated, are trained to make the sugar test of the urine. It is the duty of everyone of these to examine the other members of their families at frequent intervals. Why not teach this simple test to the students in the classes in chemistry in our high schools and urge them to keep a watch on the members of their families? Every druggist certainly should be familiar with the test and should be willing to make it on request, for a nominal fee.

It makes a great deal of difference whether a patient comes to the doctor early or late. With the better methods of treatment, the earliest cases are being arrested, if not cured. Some of them may be cured. It is still too soon to know. There is little hope of strengthening a severely weakened pancreas, or of accomplishing curative results in patients who have had the disease very long.

Treatment.—The treatment of the patient is based on certain principles which follow logically from the foregoing about the nature of the disease.

Principles guiding treatment.—If diabetes is due, as seems most likely, to the overstrain of a pancreas weak by heredity, the obvious way to manage it is to reduce the strain. This is exactly the same principle that guides us in treating heart disease. Physical rest accomplishes wonders for the heart. Careful dieting does the same for the pancreas. By so arranging the diet that the total amount of sugar, that is, the load on the pancreas, is reduced, we accomplish, first, the disappearance of sugar from the urine, second, its decrease in the blood, third, the control of annoying symptoms, such as excessive urination, excessive thirst, and dryness and itching of the skin. Simultaneously, we give the pancreas a chance to pick up and regain some strength.

In mild cases of diabetes the results obtainable by diet are entirely satisfactory and the milder the case the less the food restriction necessary. In severe cases of diabetes the dietary treatment alone is less satisfactory because the diet has to be cut so low that the patient is improperly nourished. Before the discovery of insulin was made, every such case presented a bitter dilemma. Either the diet was restricted to the point where the patient literally starved to death, or the patient could be fed; but, in that case, death from diabetic coma was to be anticipated. It is in such cases, particularly, that insulin is proving a boon. With insulin at our disposal, cases of severe diabetes can be converted into mild cases. All that is necessary is to give enough extra insulin every day to raise the patient's tolerance for sugar, and then, with a careful but adequate diet, he can enjoy normal strength and health and carry on with his usual occupation. This is not curing diabetes, but it is eliminating the worst of its terrors.

The diet can not be disregarded.—Some persons may ask why dieting is necessary with insulin? If, as seems true, the only metabolic disturbance in diabetes is a lack of sufficient insulin, then we should be able to correct this fault completely by giving sufficient insulin, and to eat what we want. This may be sound, theoretically, but is impractical for the following reason.

An uncontrolled normal diet contains approximately 300 grams, or 10 ounces of carbohydrate, 150 grams, or 5 ounces of protein, and 90 grams, or 3 ounces of fat. In the course of assimilation, about 400 grams of sugar are derived therefrom, and, to metabolize such an amount of sugar, 150 to

300 units of insulin must be necessary. A normal person probably makes, in his pancreas, 200 or 300 units of insulin a day, which is sufficient for any normal demand, but this natural insulin is doled out to his tissues, a bit at a time, so that there is never an excess of insulin in the blood.

Excessive insulin harmful.—In severe diabetes the pancreas manufactures very little insulin, not more than 20 or 30 units, and the balance necessary for the day's work must be given by hypodermic syringe in two or three doses. If the total amount of extra insulin necessary daily were 150 units, each hypodermic injection would be 50 units, and it is difficult to give such large doses as this without causing a temporary excess of insulin in the blood. Unfortunately, excessive insulin is as disagreeable as inadequate insulin. When too much insulin is present in the blood, the blood sugar falls to very low levels and a reaction occurs with symptoms that may be alarming, and results that may be serious. Consequently, very large single doses of insulin must be avoided and the total amount of sugar entering the body daily must be measured and made to balance with the insulin doses. This means dieting.

Furthermore, it proves to be very difficult to keep the level of the blood sugar low with insulin when diets are very rich in carbohydrate. The normal sugar level, as I have said, is 0.1 per cent. In uncontrolled diabetic conditions, it may be found as high as 0.5 per cent, or higher. This can be reduced by an insulin injection, but as soon as food rich in carbohydrate is eaten, back comes the sugar to a high level. In order to rest the pancreas, the blood sugar must be kept low, which can only be accomplished when the diet contains relatively little carbohydrate.

THE DIET

C *alories and sugar should be low.* —All of the principal authorities on diabetes are agreed that a diabetic patient must not overeat and become fat. In other words, the total amount of food energy, that is, calories, must be limited. All are agreed also that the diet must be kept low in sugar producing foods. This means little carbohydrate and little protein. The diet in health, as I have said, includes a great deal of carbohydrate, probably more than is wise even for perfectly normal persons. The diet in diabetes must get more of its calories from fat and less from the starches and meats. Authorities are furthermore agreed that an excessive restriction of carbohydrate (sugar and starch) may be dangerous, because with such very low carbohydrate diets the fats may fail to be properly assimilated, with resulting acid poisoning.

The authorities agree on general principles. —The actual procedures in diet-planning employed by various authorities differ but little, and only as to details. Doctor Allen, for instance, believes in much greater restriction of total food than do others. Doctor Joslin also favors rather low total food amounts and disbelieves in allowing much fat unless rather large amounts of carbohydrate can be taken. Doctor Woodyat of Chicago, the doctors in the Toronto Clinic, and Doctor McCann at the University of Rochester, New York, plan their diets in such a way that approximately one part of carbohydrate will be taken for every two and one-half parts of fat. Professor Petren of Lund, Sweden, now the leading authority in Europe, and Doctor Newburgh and Doctor Marsh of the University of Michigan, believe that restricting protein is of extreme importance, and that if this is done acidosis can be avoided even when larger proportions of fat are fed. In the Mayo Clinic, the practice is to limit protein rigidly and to limit carbohydrate rather more strictly than is done elsewhere, making the diet consist to a greater extent of fat, but planning this so that the total energy of the daily food supply will meet quite closely actual energy requirements. The procedures for arriving at these several diets can be found in various manuals that have been written for patients.

Books on diabetes for patients.—Doctor Joslin's "Diabetic Manual," Lea and Febiger, is one of these. Doctor Petty's "Diabetes, Its Treatment by Insulin and Diet," F. A. Davis Company, Philadelphia, is another. Wilder, Foley and Ellithorpe's "A Primer for Diabetic Patients," W. B. Saunders Company, Philadelphia, may be consulted for more complete descriptions of the methods employed in the Mayo Clinic than can be given here.

Patients must be trained.—The results of accurate management are so encouraging that they are almost as good as cures. They are not cures, because the fundamental island weakness is rarely if ever completely corrected, and treatment must continue for month after month. Success, therefore, rests largely in the patient's hands and the doctors' most important task is teaching the patient all that he can be taught about his diet and about the use of insulin. The books mentioned were written to help in this training of patients. In various clinics over the country, patients attend classes and are instructed in the subject of dietetics until they can weigh food and plan meals accurately so that each will contain a set number of calories and yield to the metabolism a predetermined amount of sugar. The hospital management of a case of diabetes is not complete until the patient can live a healthy life in spite of his disease. He may arrive at the hospital in a state of coma and be dragged from the very jaws of death with insulin, but afterwards, when he goes home, unless he has learned how to continue the use of insulin and combine with it an accurate diet, he will slip again into the same dangerous predicament.

It is best always to start treatment in a hospital where a systematic course of instruction can be obtained. Unfortunately, we have no schools for diabetic patients other than the hospitals, and some persons dislike hospitals. Good results can be obtained at home, provided one has the good fortune to consult a physician who will take the time to give this training. What are the essentials?

What the patient must know.—First, a knowledge of how to read food tables and, with their aid, to plan accurate diets. Food tables are lists of foods showing the composition of each, in protein, carbohydrate and fat. The books mentioned here all contain such lists. The most complete table is that published by the United States Department of Agriculture, Bulletin No. 28, "The Chemical Composition of American Food Materials," a pamphlet that may be had from the Superintendent of Documents, Government Printing Office, Washington, D. C., for the small sum of ten cents.

Second, instruction in the manner of injecting insulin, that is, in the use of the hypodermic syringe. Insulin, as has been stated, must be given hypodermically, under the skin. The technic is not difficult, but sterile precautions must be observed in order to avoid introducing disease germs with the insulin.

Third, instruction in how to test the urine for sugar. This is a simple task but of great importance. Sugar in the urine is the first signal of inadequate treatment. To postpone correcting the mistake until other signs appear such as thirst, excessive urination, and loss of strength, is to court disaster. The sugar test can be completed in three minutes, and should be made every day, preferably on a specimen of urine passed just before the patient retires for the night. This specimen should be sugar-free. If it is not, more insulin is needed or the diet requires readjustment.

Fourth, advice concerning how to meet certain complications which I shall discuss later.

TREATMENT IN CASES OF MILD DIABETES

There are instances of patients with diabetes who have lived for twenty years or more without any effort at treatment. This consoling thought must not make unwary the patient with a moderately severe or severe form of the disease. It is safer to overrate the seriousness of the condition than to commit an irreparable blunder and neglect the careful management of a serious condition. Children and young adults, for instance, may seem well during the first year after the appearance of sugar, but with few exceptions they develop the severest form of the disease later unless they are very carefully treated from the first.

A good many older persons may be treated satisfactorily with much less dietary restriction than is necessary in the severe cases. When this is possible, insulin is not needed and should not be used, or, in other words, if a condition is serious enough to require insulin, it is serious enough to require an accurately weighed diet. Occasionally patients have so little intelligence that it is hopeless to expect them to carry on the weighed diet in their homes. For such, and also for patients with very mild diabetes, the following general advice is usually beneficial:

1. Avoid sugar and all foods made with sugar, such as candy, jelly, marmalade, syrup and molasses, pies, cakes, puddings and pastries. Saccharin may be used if desired: one-fourth grain saccharin will equal one teaspoonful of sugar in sweetening value.

2. Avoid cereals (breakfast foods) and cereal products, such as mush, macaroni, spaghetti and noodles.

3. Use bread only in very small amounts, not over one ounce at a meal. Whole wheat or white breads are preferable to any so-called diabetic breads. Gluten bread, brown bread and corn bread vary widely in compositions and it is safer to avoid them.

4. Potatoes, bananas, apples, peas, dried beans, carrots, beets, turnips and onions should be used in small quantities, and not oftener than once a day.

5. Dried fruits should be avoided. Use fresh fruits whenever possible. Fruits canned without sugar are permissible. They may be purchased on the market or prepared at home. Fruits may be taken every day as substitutes for other desserts.

6. Vegetables that grow above the ground, except peas and dried beans, should be eaten in quantities sufficient to avoid hunger. Three ordinary servings of these vegetables may be included in each meal. Canned vegetables are palatable and wholesome. Fresh vegetables are, however, preferable.

7. Meat and eggs should be eaten sparingly. As much harm may result from excessive protein as from excessive carbohydrate. The diet for the day should never contain more than 60 grams (2 ounces) of lean meat, weighed cooked, and three eggs. Thirty grams (1 ounce) of bacon, weighed cooked, may be included. Meat includes chicken, game, and fish.

8. Fats, including butter or oleomargarine, nut butter, bacon fat, olive oil, Wesson oil, or other salad oil may be eaten freely.

9. Cream is a very useful food for diabetic patients, and may be taken freely. Milk is relatively high in carbohydrate and less nutritious.

10. The amount of fat, such as butter or cream, should be adjusted so as to provide adequate, but not excessive, nutrition. A rising body-weight calls for less food and, under such circumstances,

the amount of fat should be reduced.

11. Coffee and tea should be used sparingly, not in excess of one cupful of either at each meal.

12. Condiments, such as salt, pepper and vinegar, may be used in reasonable amount.

If sugar appears in the urine, bread should be omitted. If it persists after thus reducing the carbohydrate intake, the condition of the patient is severe enough to warrant instituting the more accurate management discussed herein.

THE TREATMENT OF FEVERS OCCURRING IN DIABETIC PATIENTS

*F**evers increase the need for insulin.*—Today, with insulin, a properly dieted patient is as robust and capable as his normal neighbor. His handicap is the continued necessity for keeping his enemy under control, but if this control is watchfully maintained, he should live as long and as useful a life as do his fellows. However, throughout his life he is exposed, as are his fellows, to diseases other than diabetes. Measles, mumps, scarlet fever, diphtheria, acute colds, influenza, pneumonia, and other germ diseases, the so-called infectious diseases, will attack him, and when they do they invariably aggravate his diabetes and, by preventing the utilization of his sugars, subject him to the danger of acid poisoning from smoldering fats. Therefore, when such complications occur, a patient must have insulin, whether he has been able to do without it before or not, and usually the doses necessary to control these critical emergencies must be large. For instance, a patient on a set diet, whose urine remains free from sugar with 20 units of insulin, may require 40 units daily whenever he takes cold. A serious infection like pneumonia may make it necessary to use 80 units of insulin daily. Under normal circumstances, a patient taking 20 or 30 units of insulin daily, does very well when this is divided into two doses of 15 units each, and one dose is injected before breakfast, and the second before the evening meal. During an attack of pneumonia or any other fever-producing complication, it may be necessary to resort to four injections, spaced at six-hour intervals. It is usually necessary to modify and reduce the diet when a patient is sick. It is always wise to eat less. In particular, the fat allowance of the diet should be reduced. It is wise not to reduce the carbohydrate. The patient with fever may be nauseated during the course of a fever and refuse all food. Under such circumstances, less insulin may be required; usually, however, large doses are still necessary. The reason for this is not clear, but apparently the poisons created in the course of germ diseases counteract the effect of insulin. During disease, the urine should be examined every six hours and the dose of insulin necessary may be judged from the amount of sugar found.

OPERATIONS ON DIABETIC PATIENTS

Special precautions necessary in operating on diabetic patients.—It is self-evident that a person with diabetes is no less likely to develop appendicitis, gallstones, or cancer than he would be without diabetes. Consequently, serious operations are occasionally necessary. The danger from such procedures is many times greater in diabetic patients than in others, unless the diabetes is closely controlled. Formerly one out of every three operations on diabetic patients terminated fatally. This was because the anesthetic, ether or chloroform, provoked acid poisoning, and because the enfeebled patient was little prepared to withstand the shock of loss of blood, and injury. The added danger of diabetes may be avoided if the patient is in good condition before he goes to operation, and if acidosis is promptly combated with insulin. It is wise for the diabetic patient to employ only a very skillful surgeon, and to make certain either that he is familiar with the treatment of diabetes, or that he has associated with him some physician who has had a considerable experience with diabetes.

MISCELLANEOUS COMPLICATIONS

*A*rteriosclerosis.—When we pass the age of thirty-eight, we are enjoying life which was denied our grandparents. The expectancy of life for a newborn baby in 1860 was thirty-eight years. Now it is nearly sixty years. This accounts, in a large measure, for the specially rapid increase in the amount of diabetes among people more than forty-five, and for the larger incidence today of other diseases of a chronic type. Hardening of the arteries, or arteriosclerosis, is a complication with which older diabetic patients are frequently afflicted. As has been said, arteriosclerosis may be a cause of diabetes in a predisposed person, but be that as it may, diabetes, once established, unless controlled, aggravates and intensifies disease of the arteries. It is, therefore, important for the older diabetic patient to make a serious effort to avoid arteriosclerosis by keeping his diabetes checked. Most of the complications which harass and endanger the older patient are due to hardening of the arteries. In this disease, the elastic contracting tissue in the hollow muscular tubes that carry blood is replaced, bit by bit, with scar tissue.

Apoplexy, heart trouble, gangrene.—The walls of the tubes thicken, become brittle, and what results? A vessel in the brain breaks, and hemorrhage in the brain may cause apoplexy. A vessel may also break in the eye. The amount of blood that can pass through the narrowed tubes is too little to supply the beating heart, and pain results, called angina, or irregular heart action or even heart failure. The circulation in the legs is restricted, and pains result, and sometimes gangrene. Coma, it will be remembered, is the chief cause of death among younger diabetic patients. Coma can now be prevented and no one should die from coma. Gangrene is the chief cause of death among older patients. In gangrene, usually of the legs, the tissues lose their vitality because of lack of blood; infection follows and blood poisoning results.

Prevent gangrene.—We must prevent these deaths from gangrene. It can be done by watchfulness and attention. Keeping the urine sugar-free is the first requisite. Gangrenous ulcers of the feet can be made to heal by vigorous treatment with insulin, and diet. It is of great importance to encourage the circulation in the feet by massage and proper exercises. Finally, care in avoiding bruises and cuts of the skin of the feet will prevent much trouble. Every old diabetic patient should wash his feet daily, wear clean stockings, and very comfortable shoes. Watch and guard the feet. Achilles, the Greek hero, must have been a diabetic. The only vulnerable spot on his body was his heel. When before the walls of Troy the spear of Paris touched him on the heel, he died. Watch and guard the feet.

www.ingramcontent.com/pod-product-compliance
Lightning Source LLC
Chambersburg PA
CBHW060657280326
41933CB00012B/2221